eat

drink

move

sleep

ISBN 978-1-4521-4210-4

Manufactured in China

Designed by Sara Schneider and Amanda Sim

Text by Laura Lee Mattingly

10 9 8 7 6 5 4 3 2

Chronicle Books LLC
680 Second Street
San Francisco, California 94107
www.chroniclebooks.com

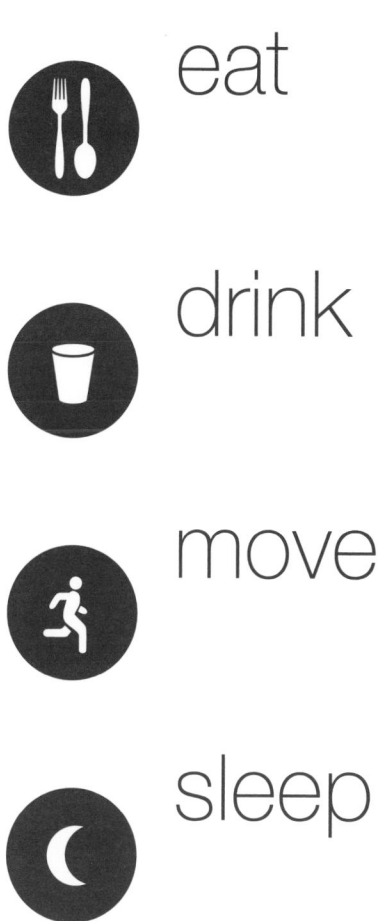

eat

drink

move

sleep

a health tracking journal

CHRONICLE BOOKS

SAN FRANCISCO

Be Better. Every Day.

You know what you need to do. Get eight hours of sleep. Drink plenty of water. Move your body every day. Eat nourishing foods. Minimize vices such as caffeine, sugar, and alcohol. You know this, but of course it's all too easy to forget while in the whirlwind of your daily routine. Goals go out the window and suddenly weeks have passed since you last exercised and you're groggy from lack of sleep and you're so stressed out you're just going to order pizza for dinner tonight, okay?

We've all been there.

This journal is here to help. There are no diet plans or wellness doctrines in these pages. You've read the articles and seen the news stories. It's not knowledge you're lacking—it's time. And maybe some focus.

Just as keeping a budget leads to improved financial stability, logging your daily health practices will lead to sustained well-being. This journal focuses on four cornerstones of health: diet, exercise, sleep, and mental balance. Each day, record what you ate, the amount of water you drank, how you exercised, the hours you've slept, and what you did for your mind and stress level. There is also an "other" category where you can track whatever you may be focusing on that week—be it weight, sugar, or calories, plus space for making weekly goals. Use this journal to track your health for thirty weeks, or for a few weeks at a time whenever you need to reset. The charts are general on purpose, because the specifics are up to you.

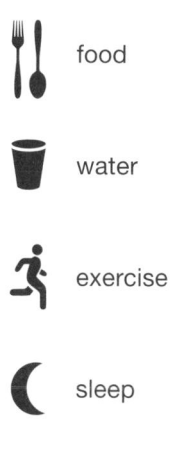

food

water

exercise

sleep

stress relief and mental balance

As you fill out the pages and keep a record of your daily habits, you will likely surprise yourself. Maybe you're sleeping better than you thought. Or you're exercising way less than you thought. Perhaps all those midday coffee runs are adding up to too much caffeine. Seeing your own health patterns will help you focus more on certain areas as needed and show you where you're already taking steps to improve your health.

The simple act of filling out this journal will motivate you to do as much as you can for your health every day. And shouldn't that be the ultimate goal?

WEEK OF :   /   /   —   /   /

GOALS :

_____

_____

_____

Monday

Date   /   /

🍴				
	Breakfast	🥤 Water		oz/ml
	Lunch	🏃 Exercise		
	Dinner	🌙 Sleep	h	m
	Snacks	🧘 Stress Relief		

Other _____

Tuesday

Date   /   /

🍴				
	Breakfast	🥤 Water		oz/ml
	Lunch	🏃 Exercise		
	Dinner	🌙 Sleep	h	m
	Snacks	🧘 Stress Relief		

Other _____

Wednesday

Date   /   /

🍴			🗑		
	Breakfast		Water		oz/ml
	Lunch		🏃 Exercise		
	Dinner		🌙 Sleep	h	m
	Snacks		🧘 Stress Relief		

Other

Thursday

Date   /   /

🍴			🗑		
	Breakfast		Water		oz/ml
	Lunch		🏃 Exercise		
	Dinner		🌙 Sleep	h	m
	Snacks		🧘 Stress Relief		

Other

Friday

Date   /   /

🍴			🗑		
	Breakfast		Water		oz/ml
	Lunch		🏃 Exercise		
	Dinner		🌙 Sleep	h	m
	Snacks		🧘 Stress Relief		

Other

Saturday

Date   /   /

Breakfast	Water	oz/ml
Lunch	Exercise	
Dinner	Sleep h m	
Snacks	Stress Relief	

Other

Sunday

Date   /   /

Breakfast	Water	oz/ml
Lunch	Exercise	
Dinner	Sleep h m	
Snacks	Stress Relief	

Other

How am I feeling physically and mentally?

Challenges?

Achievements?

WEEK OF :   /   /   —   /   /

GOALS :

Monday
Date   /   /

🍴	Breakfast	🗑 Water	oz/ml
	Lunch	🏃 Exercise	
	Dinner	🌙 Sleep	h m
	Snacks	🧘 Stress Relief	

Other

Tuesday
Date   /   /

🍴	Breakfast	🗑 Water	oz/ml
	Lunch	🏃 Exercise	
	Dinner	🌙 Sleep	h m
	Snacks	🧘 Stress Relief	

Other

Wednesday

Date   /   /

Breakfast		Water	oz/ml
Lunch		Exercise	
Dinner		Sleep	h m
Snacks		Stress Relief	

Other

Thursday

Date   /   /

Breakfast		Water	oz/ml
Lunch		Exercise	
Dinner		Sleep	h m
Snacks		Stress Relief	

Other

Friday

Date   /   /

Breakfast		Water	oz/ml
Lunch		Exercise	
Dinner		Sleep	h m
Snacks		Stress Relief	

Other

Saturday

Date   /   /

🍴	Breakfast	🗑 Water	oz/ml
	Lunch	🏃 Exercise	
	Dinner	🌙 Sleep h m	
	Snacks	🧘 Stress Relief	

Other

Sunday

Date   /   /

🍴	Breakfast	🗑 Water	oz/ml
	Lunch	🏃 Exercise	
	Dinner	🌙 Sleep h m	
	Snacks	🧘 Stress Relief	

Other

How am I feeling physically and mentally?

_____

_____

_____

_____

_____

_____

Challenges?

_____

_____

_____

_____

_____

_____

Achievements?

_____

_____

_____

_____

_____

_____

WEEK OF : / / — / /

GOALS :
_____
_____
_____

Monday   Date   /   /

🍴 Breakfast

Lunch

Dinner

Snacks

🥤 Water   oz/ml

🏃 Exercise

🌙 Sleep   h   m

🧘 Stress Relief

Other _____

Tuesday   Date   /   /

🍴 Breakfast

Lunch

Dinner

Snacks

🥤 Water   oz/ml

🏃 Exercise

🌙 Sleep   h   m

🧘 Stress Relief

Other _____

Wednesday

Date   /   /

🍴 Breakfast		🥤 Water	oz/ml
Lunch		🏃 Exercise	
Dinner		🌙 Sleep	h m
Snacks		🧘 Stress Relief	

Other

Thursday

Date   /   /

🍴 Breakfast		🥤 Water	oz/ml
Lunch		🏃 Exercise	
Dinner		🌙 Sleep	h m
Snacks		🧘 Stress Relief	

Other

Friday

Date   /   /

🍴 Breakfast		🥤 Water	oz/ml
Lunch		🏃 Exercise	
Dinner		🌙 Sleep	h m
Snacks		🧘 Stress Relief	

Other

Saturday

Date   /   /

Breakfast	Water	oz/ml
Lunch	Exercise	
Dinner	Sleep	h m
Snacks	Stress Relief	

Other _____

Sunday

Date   /   /

Breakfast	Water	oz/ml
Lunch	Exercise	
Dinner	Sleep	h m
Snacks	Stress Relief	

Other _____

How am I feeling physically and mentally?

Challenges?

Achievements?

WEEK OF :   /   /   —   /   /

GOALS :

_____

_____

_____

Monday
Date   /   /

Breakfast	Water	oz/ml
Lunch	Exercise	
Dinner	Sleep	h m
Snacks	Stress Relief	

Other _____

Tuesday
Date   /   /

Breakfast	Water	oz/ml
Lunch	Exercise	
Dinner	Sleep	h m
Snacks	Stress Relief	

Other _____

Wednesday

Date   /   /

🍴			
	Breakfast	🗑 Water	oz/ml
	Lunch	🏃 Exercise	
	Dinner	🌙 Sleep h m	
	Snacks	🧘 Stress Relief	

Other _____

Thursday

Date   /   /

🍴			
	Breakfast	🗑 Water	oz/ml
	Lunch	🏃 Exercise	
	Dinner	🌙 Sleep h m	
	Snacks	🧘 Stress Relief	

Other _____

Friday

Date   /   /

🍴			
	Breakfast	🗑 Water	oz/ml
	Lunch	🏃 Exercise	
	Dinner	🌙 Sleep h m	
	Snacks	🧘 Stress Relief	

Other _____

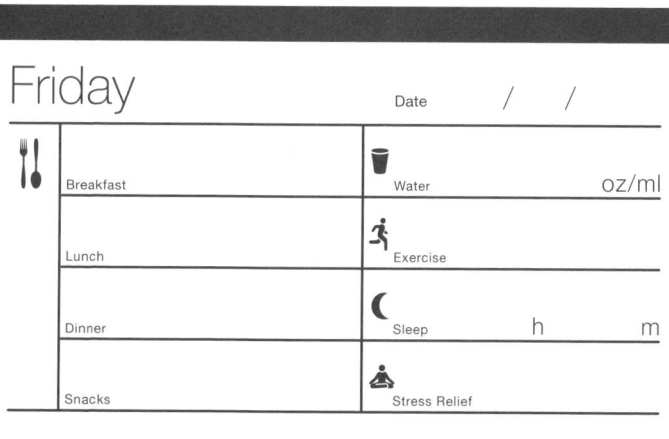

Saturday

Date   /   /

Breakfast	Water oz/ml
Lunch	Exercise
Dinner	Sleep h m
Snacks	Stress Relief

Other

Sunday

Date   /   /

Breakfast	Water oz/ml
Lunch	Exercise
Dinner	Sleep h m
Snacks	Stress Relief

Other

How am I feeling physically and mentally?

Challenges?

Achievements?

WEEK OF :   /   /   —   /   /

GOALS :
_____
_____
_____

Monday   Date   /   /

Breakfast		Water	oz/ml
Lunch		Exercise	
Dinner		Sleep	h m
Snacks		Stress Relief	

Other _____

Tuesday   Date   /   /

Breakfast		Water	oz/ml
Lunch		Exercise	
Dinner		Sleep	h m
Snacks		Stress Relief	

Other _____

Wednesday

Date   /   /

🍴			
	Breakfast	🗑 Water	oz/ml
	Lunch	🏃 Exercise	
	Dinner	🌙 Sleep	h m
	Snacks	🧘 Stress Relief	

Other _____

Thursday

Date   /   /

🍴			
	Breakfast	🗑 Water	oz/ml
	Lunch	🏃 Exercise	
	Dinner	🌙 Sleep	h m
	Snacks	🧘 Stress Relief	

Other _____

Friday

Date   /   /

🍴			
	Breakfast	🗑 Water	oz/ml
	Lunch	🏃 Exercise	
	Dinner	🌙 Sleep	h m
	Snacks	🧘 Stress Relief	

Other _____

Saturday

Date   /   /

🍴		🗑	
Breakfast		Water	oz/ml
Lunch		Exercise	
Dinner		Sleep	h m
Snacks		Stress Relief	

Other _____

Sunday

Date   /   /

🍴		🗑	
Breakfast		Water	oz/ml
Lunch		Exercise	
Dinner		Sleep	h m
Snacks		Stress Relief	

Other _____

How am I feeling physically and mentally?

_____

_____

_____

_____

_____

_____

Challenges?

_____

_____

_____

_____

_____

_____

Achievements?

_____

_____

_____

_____

_____

_____

WEEK OF : / / — / /

GOALS :
_____
_____
_____

Monday
Date / /

🍴 Breakfast

Lunch

Dinner

Snacks

🥤 Water _____ oz/ml

🏃 Exercise

🌙 Sleep ___ h ___ m

🧘 Stress Relief

Other _____

Tuesday
Date / /

🍴 Breakfast

Lunch

Dinner

Snacks

🥤 Water _____ oz/ml

🏃 Exercise

🌙 Sleep ___ h ___ m

🧘 Stress Relief

Other _____

Wednesday

Date ___ / ___ / ___

🍴			
	Breakfast	🗑 Water	oz/ml
	Lunch	🏃 Exercise	
	Dinner	🌙 Sleep	h m
	Snacks	🧘 Stress Relief	

Other _____

Thursday

Date ___ / ___ / ___

🍴			
	Breakfast	🗑 Water	oz/ml
	Lunch	🏃 Exercise	
	Dinner	🌙 Sleep	h m
	Snacks	🧘 Stress Relief	

Other _____

Friday

Date ___ / ___ / ___

🍴			
	Breakfast	🗑 Water	oz/ml
	Lunch	🏃 Exercise	
	Dinner	🌙 Sleep	h m
	Snacks	🧘 Stress Relief	

Other _____

Saturday

Date   /   /

Breakfast	Water oz/ml
Lunch	Exercise
Dinner	Sleep h m
Snacks	Stress Relief

Other

Sunday

Date   /   /

Breakfast	Water oz/ml
Lunch	Exercise
Dinner	Sleep h m
Snacks	Stress Relief

Other

How am I feeling physically and mentally?

_____

_____

_____

_____

_____

_____

Challenges?

_____

_____

_____

_____

_____

_____

Achievements?

_____

_____

_____

_____

_____

_____

WEEK OF : / / — / /

GOALS :
_____
_____
_____

Monday
Date / /

🍴	Breakfast		🗑	Water	oz/ml
	Lunch		🏃	Exercise	
	Dinner		🌙	Sleep	h m
	Snacks		🧘	Stress Relief	

Other _____

Tuesday
Date / /

🍴	Breakfast		🗑	Water	oz/ml
	Lunch		🏃	Exercise	
	Dinner		🌙	Sleep	h m
	Snacks		🧘	Stress Relief	

Other _____

Wednesday

Date   /   /

Breakfast	Water oz/ml
Lunch	Exercise
Dinner	Sleep h m
Snacks	Stress Relief

Other

Thursday

Date   /   /

Breakfast	Water oz/ml
Lunch	Exercise
Dinner	Sleep h m
Snacks	Stress Relief

Other

Friday

Date   /   /

Breakfast	Water oz/ml
Lunch	Exercise
Dinner	Sleep h m
Snacks	Stress Relief

Other

Saturday

Date   /   /

🍴		🗑	
	Breakfast		Water oz/ml
	Lunch	🏃 Exercise	
	Dinner	🌙 Sleep h m	
	Snacks	🧘 Stress Relief	

Other

Sunday

Date   /   /

🍴		🗑	
	Breakfast		Water oz/ml
	Lunch	🏃 Exercise	
	Dinner	🌙 Sleep h m	
	Snacks	🧘 Stress Relief	

Other

How am I feeling physically and mentally?

Challenges?

Achievements?

WEEK OF :   /   /   —   /   /

GOALS :
_____
_____
_____

Monday   Date   /   /

🍴	Breakfast		🗑 Water		oz/ml
	Lunch		🏃 Exercise		
	Dinner		🌙 Sleep	h	m
	Snacks		🧘 Stress Relief		

Other _____

Tuesday   Date   /   /

🍴	Breakfast		🗑 Water		oz/ml
	Lunch		🏃 Exercise		
	Dinner		🌙 Sleep	h	m
	Snacks		🧘 Stress Relief		

Other _____

Wednesday

Date   /   /

🍴	Breakfast	🗑 Water	oz/ml
	Lunch	🏃 Exercise	
	Dinner	🌙 Sleep	h m
	Snacks	🧘 Stress Relief	

Other

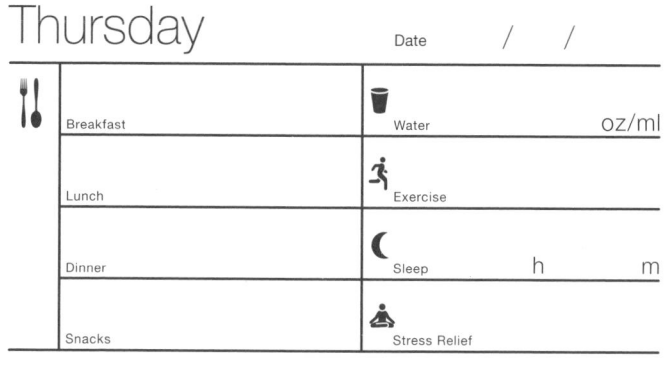

Thursday

Date   /   /

🍴	Breakfast	🗑 Water	oz/ml
	Lunch	🏃 Exercise	
	Dinner	🌙 Sleep	h m
	Snacks	🧘 Stress Relief	

Other

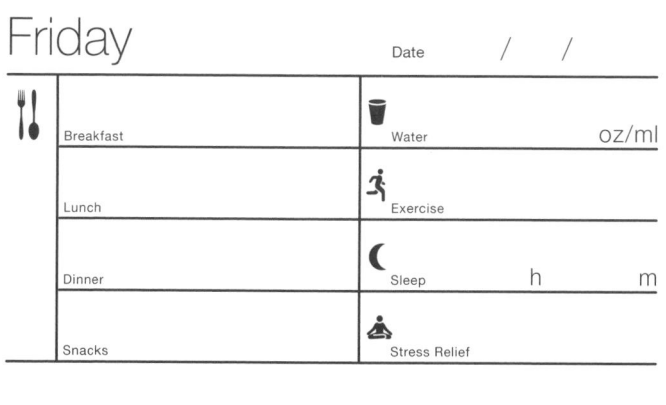

Friday

Date   /   /

🍴	Breakfast	🗑 Water	oz/ml
	Lunch	🏃 Exercise	
	Dinner	🌙 Sleep	h m
	Snacks	🧘 Stress Relief	

Other

Saturday

Date   /   /

Breakfast	Water oz/ml
Lunch	Exercise
Dinner	Sleep h m
Snacks	Stress Relief

Other

Sunday

Date   /   /

Breakfast	Water oz/ml
Lunch	Exercise
Dinner	Sleep h m
Snacks	Stress Relief

Other

How am I feeling physically and mentally?

_____

_____

_____

_____

_____

_____

Challenges?

_____

_____

_____

_____

_____

_____

Achievements?

_____

_____

_____

_____

_____

_____

WEEK OF :   /   /   —   /   /

GOALS :
_____
_____
_____

Monday   Date   /   /

Breakfast	Water oz/ml
Lunch	Exercise
Dinner	Sleep h m
Snacks	Stress Relief

Other _____

Tuesday   Date   /   /

Breakfast	Water oz/ml
Lunch	Exercise
Dinner	Sleep h m
Snacks	Stress Relief

Other _____

Wednesday

Date   /   /

Breakfast		Water	oz/ml
Lunch		Exercise	
Dinner		Sleep	h m
Snacks		Stress Relief	

Other _____

Thursday

Date   /   /

Breakfast		Water	oz/ml
Lunch		Exercise	
Dinner		Sleep	h m
Snacks		Stress Relief	

Other _____

Friday

Date   /   /

Breakfast		Water	oz/ml
Lunch		Exercise	
Dinner		Sleep	h m
Snacks		Stress Relief	

Other _____

Saturday

Date   /   /

Breakfast	Water		oz/ml
Lunch	Exercise		
Dinner	Sleep	h	m
Snacks	Stress Relief		

Other

Sunday

Date   /   /

Breakfast	Water		oz/ml
Lunch	Exercise		
Dinner	Sleep	h	m
Snacks	Stress Relief		

Other

How am I feeling physically and mentally?

Challenges?

Achievements?

WEEK OF :   /   /   —   /   /

GOALS :

_____

_____

Monday

Date   /   /

Breakfast	Water	oz/ml
Lunch	Exercise	
Dinner	Sleep h m	
Snacks	Stress Relief	

Other

Tuesday

Date   /   /

Breakfast	Water	oz/ml
Lunch	Exercise	
Dinner	Sleep h m	
Snacks	Stress Relief	

Other

Wednesday

Date   /   /

Breakfast		Water	oz/ml
Lunch		Exercise	
Dinner		Sleep	h m
Snacks		Stress Relief	

Other _____

Thursday

Date   /   /

Breakfast		Water	oz/ml
Lunch		Exercise	
Dinner		Sleep	h m
Snacks		Stress Relief	

Other _____

Friday

Date   /   /

Breakfast		Water	oz/ml
Lunch		Exercise	
Dinner		Sleep	h m
Snacks		Stress Relief	

Other _____

Saturday

Date   /   /

Breakfast	Water	oz/ml
Lunch	Exercise	
Dinner	Sleep	h m
Snacks	Stress Relief	

Other

Sunday

Date   /   /

Breakfast	Water	oz/ml
Lunch	Exercise	
Dinner	Sleep	h m
Snacks	Stress Relief	

Other

How am I feeling physically and mentally?

_____

_____

_____

_____

_____

_____

Challenges?

_____

_____

_____

_____

_____

_____

Achievements?

_____

_____

_____

_____

_____

_____

WEEK OF : / / — / /

GOALS :
_____
_____
_____

Monday

Date / /

Breakfast		Water	oz/ml
Lunch		Exercise	
Dinner		Sleep	h	m
Snacks		Stress Relief	

Other _____

Tuesday

Date / /

Breakfast		Water	oz/ml
Lunch		Exercise	
Dinner		Sleep	h	m
Snacks		Stress Relief	

Other _____

Wednesday

Date ___ / ___ / ___

🍴			
Breakfast		🗑 Water	oz/ml
Lunch		🏃 Exercise	
Dinner		🌙 Sleep	h m
Snacks		🧘 Stress Relief	

Other _____

Thursday

Date ___ / ___ / ___

🍴			
Breakfast		🗑 Water	oz/ml
Lunch		🏃 Exercise	
Dinner		🌙 Sleep	h m
Snacks		🧘 Stress Relief	

Other _____

Friday

Date ___ / ___ / ___

🍴			
Breakfast		🗑 Water	oz/ml
Lunch		🏃 Exercise	
Dinner		🌙 Sleep	h m
Snacks		🧘 Stress Relief	

Other _____

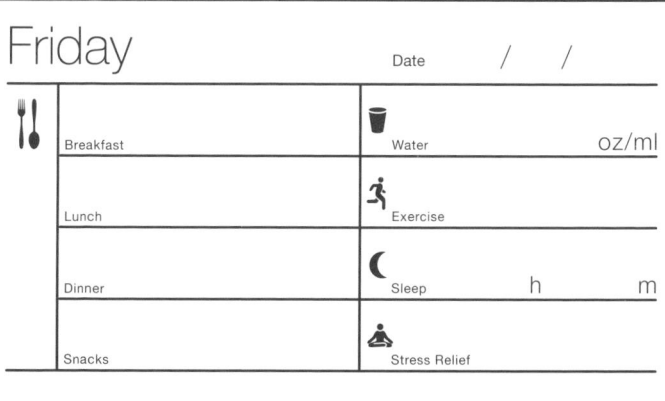

Saturday

Date   /   /

Breakfast		Water	oz/ml
Lunch		Exercise	
Dinner		Sleep	h m
Snacks		Stress Relief	

Other

Sunday

Date   /   /

Breakfast		Water	oz/ml
Lunch		Exercise	
Dinner		Sleep	h m
Snacks		Stress Relief	

Other

How am I feeling physically and mentally?

_____

_____

_____

_____

_____

_____

Challenges?

_____

_____

_____

_____

_____

_____

Achievements?

_____

_____

_____

_____

_____

_____

WEEK OF :   /   /   —   /   /

GOALS :

_____

_____

_____

Monday

Date   /   /

🍴				
	Breakfast	🗑 Water		oz/ml
	Lunch	🏃 Exercise		
	Dinner	🌙 Sleep	h	m
	Snacks	🧘 Stress Relief		

Other _____

Tuesday

Date   /   /

🍴				
	Breakfast	🗑 Water		oz/ml
	Lunch	🏃 Exercise		
	Dinner	🌙 Sleep	h	m
	Snacks	🧘 Stress Relief		

Other _____

Wednesday

Date   /   /

🍴			Water	oz/ml
	Breakfast			
	Lunch		🏃 Exercise	
	Dinner		🌙 Sleep	h m
	Snacks		🧘 Stress Relief	

Other _____

Thursday

Date   /   /

🍴			Water	oz/ml
	Breakfast			
	Lunch		🏃 Exercise	
	Dinner		🌙 Sleep	h m
	Snacks		🧘 Stress Relief	

Other _____

Friday

Date   /   /

🍴			Water	oz/ml
	Breakfast			
	Lunch		🏃 Exercise	
	Dinner		🌙 Sleep	h m
	Snacks		🧘 Stress Relief	

Other _____

Saturday

Date   /   /

🍴			
	Breakfast	🗑 Water	oz/ml
	Lunch	🏃 Exercise	
	Dinner	🌙 Sleep	h m
	Snacks	🧘 Stress Relief	

Other _____

Sunday

Date   /   /

🍴			
	Breakfast	🗑 Water	oz/ml
	Lunch	🏃 Exercise	
	Dinner	🌙 Sleep	h m
	Snacks	🧘 Stress Relief	

Other _____

How am I feeling physically and mentally?

Challenges?

Achievements?

WEEK OF : / / — / /

GOALS :
_____
_____
_____

Monday

Date / /

🍴 Breakfast

Lunch

Dinner

Snacks

🥤 Water   oz/ml

🏃 Exercise

🌙 Sleep   h   m

🧘 Stress Relief

Other _____

Tuesday

Date / /

🍴 Breakfast

Lunch

Dinner

Snacks

🥤 Water   oz/ml

🏃 Exercise

🌙 Sleep   h   m

🧘 Stress Relief

Other _____

Wednesday

Date   /   /

Breakfast	Water	oz/ml
Lunch	Exercise	
Dinner	Sleep h m	
Snacks	Stress Relief	

Other _____

Thursday

Date   /   /

Breakfast	Water	oz/ml
Lunch	Exercise	
Dinner	Sleep h m	
Snacks	Stress Relief	

Other _____

Friday

Date   /   /

Breakfast	Water	oz/ml
Lunch	Exercise	
Dinner	Sleep h m	
Snacks	Stress Relief	

Other _____

Saturday

Date   /   /

Breakfast	Water	oz/ml
Lunch	Exercise	
Dinner	Sleep	h m
Snacks	Stress Relief	

Other

Sunday

Date   /   /

Breakfast	Water	oz/ml
Lunch	Exercise	
Dinner	Sleep	h m
Snacks	Stress Relief	

Other

How am I feeling physically and mentally?

_____

_____

_____

_____

_____

_____

Challenges?

_____

_____

_____

_____

_____

Achievements?

_____

_____

_____

_____

_____

WEEK OF :   /   /   —   /   /

GOALS :
_____
_____
_____

Monday   Date   /   /

🍴			
	Breakfast	Water	oz/ml
	Lunch	Exercise	
	Dinner	Sleep h m	
	Snacks	Stress Relief	

Other _____

Tuesday   Date   /   /

🍴			
	Breakfast	Water	oz/ml
	Lunch	Exercise	
	Dinner	Sleep h m	
	Snacks	Stress Relief	

Other _____

Wednesday

Date   /   /

🍴			
	Breakfast	🗑 Water	oz/ml
	Lunch	🏃 Exercise	
	Dinner	🌙 Sleep	h m
	Snacks	🧘 Stress Relief	

Other

Thursday

Date   /   /

🍴			
	Breakfast	🗑 Water	oz/ml
	Lunch	🏃 Exercise	
	Dinner	🌙 Sleep	h m
	Snacks	🧘 Stress Relief	

Other

Friday

Date   /   /

🍴			
	Breakfast	🗑 Water	oz/ml
	Lunch	🏃 Exercise	
	Dinner	🌙 Sleep	h m
	Snacks	🧘 Stress Relief	

Other

Saturday

Date   /   /

Breakfast		Water	oz/ml
Lunch		Exercise	
Dinner		Sleep	h m
Snacks		Stress Relief	

Other

Sunday

Date   /   /

Breakfast		Water	oz/ml
Lunch		Exercise	
Dinner		Sleep	h m
Snacks		Stress Relief	

Other

How am I feeling physically and mentally?

Challenges?

Achievements?

WEEK OF :   /   /   —   /   /

GOALS :
_____
_____
_____

Monday   Date   /   /

🍴	Breakfast		🗑 Water	oz/ml
	Lunch		🏃 Exercise	
	Dinner		🌙 Sleep	h m
	Snacks		🧘 Stress Relief	

Other _____

Tuesday   Date   /   /

🍴	Breakfast		🗑 Water	oz/ml
	Lunch		🏃 Exercise	
	Dinner		🌙 Sleep	h m
	Snacks		🧘 Stress Relief	

Other _____

Wednesday

Date ___ / ___ / ___

🍴			
	Breakfast	🗑 Water	oz/ml
	Lunch	🏃 Exercise	
	Dinner	🌙 Sleep	h ___ m
	Snacks	🧘 Stress Relief	

Other _____

Thursday

Date ___ / ___ / ___

🍴			
	Breakfast	🗑 Water	oz/ml
	Lunch	🏃 Exercise	
	Dinner	🌙 Sleep	h ___ m
	Snacks	🧘 Stress Relief	

Other _____

Friday

Date ___ / ___ / ___

🍴			
	Breakfast	🗑 Water	oz/ml
	Lunch	🏃 Exercise	
	Dinner	🌙 Sleep	h ___ m
	Snacks	🧘 Stress Relief	

Other _____

Saturday

Date   /   /

🍴	Breakfast		🗑 Water	oz/ml
	Lunch		🏃 Exercise	
	Dinner		🌙 Sleep	h m
	Snacks		🧘 Stress Relief	

Other

Sunday

Date   /   /

🍴	Breakfast		🗑 Water	oz/ml
	Lunch		🏃 Exercise	
	Dinner		🌙 Sleep	h m
	Snacks		🧘 Stress Relief	

Other

How am I feeling physically and mentally?

Challenges?

Achievements?

WEEK OF :   /   /   —   /   /

GOALS :
_____
_____
_____

Monday   Date   /   /

🍴	Breakfast		🗑 Water		oz/ml
	Lunch		🏃 Exercise		
	Dinner		🌙 Sleep	h	m
	Snacks		🧘 Stress Relief		

Other

Tuesday   Date   /   /

🍴	Breakfast		🗑 Water		oz/ml
	Lunch		🏃 Exercise		
	Dinner		🌙 Sleep	h	m
	Snacks		🧘 Stress Relief		

Other

Wednesday

Date   /   /

🍴			
Breakfast		🗑 Water	oz/ml
Lunch		🏃 Exercise	
Dinner		🌙 Sleep	h m
Snacks		🧘 Stress Relief	

Other

Thursday

Date   /   /

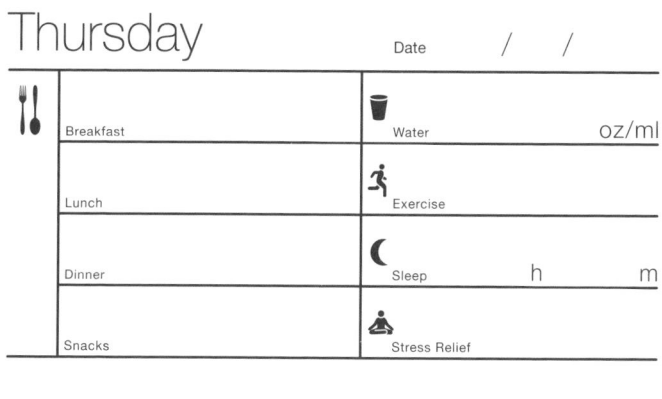

🍴			
Breakfast		🗑 Water	oz/ml
Lunch		🏃 Exercise	
Dinner		🌙 Sleep	h m
Snacks		🧘 Stress Relief	

Other

Friday

Date   /   /

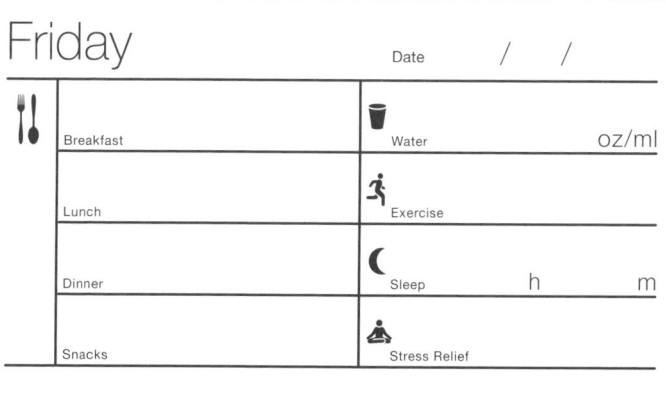

🍴			
Breakfast		🗑 Water	oz/ml
Lunch		🏃 Exercise	
Dinner		🌙 Sleep	h m
Snacks		🧘 Stress Relief	

Other

Saturday

Date   /   /

🍴		🥤 Water	oz/ml
	Breakfast		
	Lunch	🏃 Exercise	
	Dinner	🌙 Sleep	h m
	Snacks	🧘 Stress Relief	

Other

Sunday

Date   /   /

🍴		🥤 Water	oz/ml
	Breakfast		
	Lunch	🏃 Exercise	
	Dinner	🌙 Sleep	h m
	Snacks	🧘 Stress Relief	

Other

How am I feeling physically and mentally?

Challenges?

Achievements?

WEEK OF :   /   /   —   /   /

GOALS :

Monday   Date   /   /

🍴	Breakfast		🗑 Water		oz/ml
	Lunch		🏃 Exercise		
	Dinner		🌙 Sleep	h	m
	Snacks		🧘 Stress Relief		

Other

Tuesday   Date   /   /

🍴	Breakfast		🗑 Water		oz/ml
	Lunch		🏃 Exercise		
	Dinner		🌙 Sleep	h	m
	Snacks		🧘 Stress Relief		

Other

Wednesday

Date   /   /

🍴			
	Breakfast	🗑 Water	oz/ml
	Lunch	🏃 Exercise	
	Dinner	🌙 Sleep	h m
	Snacks	🧘 Stress Relief	

Other

Thursday

Date   /   /

🍴			
	Breakfast	🗑 Water	oz/ml
	Lunch	🏃 Exercise	
	Dinner	🌙 Sleep	h m
	Snacks	🧘 Stress Relief	

Other

Friday

Date   /   /

🍴			
	Breakfast	🗑 Water	oz/ml
	Lunch	🏃 Exercise	
	Dinner	🌙 Sleep	h m
	Snacks	🧘 Stress Relief	

Other

Saturday

Date   /   /

Breakfast	Water oz/ml
Lunch	Exercise
Dinner	Sleep h m
Snacks	Stress Relief

Other

Sunday

Date   /   /

Breakfast	Water oz/ml
Lunch	Exercise
Dinner	Sleep h m
Snacks	Stress Relief

Other

How am I feeling physically and mentally?

Challenges?

Achievements?

WEEK OF : / / — / /

GOALS :
_____
_____
_____

Monday
Date / /

Breakfast		Water	oz/ml
Lunch		Exercise	
Dinner		Sleep	h m
Snacks		Stress Relief	

Other _____

Tuesday
Date / /

Breakfast		Water	oz/ml
Lunch		Exercise	
Dinner		Sleep	h m
Snacks		Stress Relief	

Other _____

Wednesday

Date   /   /

🍴	Breakfast	🗑 Water		oz/ml
	Lunch	🏃 Exercise		
	Dinner	🌙 Sleep	h	m
	Snacks	🧘 Stress Relief		

Other _____

Thursday

Date   /   /

🍴	Breakfast	🗑 Water		oz/ml
	Lunch	🏃 Exercise		
	Dinner	🌙 Sleep	h	m
	Snacks	🧘 Stress Relief		

Other _____

Friday

Date   /   /

🍴	Breakfast	🗑 Water		oz/ml
	Lunch	🏃 Exercise		
	Dinner	🌙 Sleep	h	m
	Snacks	🧘 Stress Relief		

Other _____

Saturday

Date   /   /

🍴		🗑	
	Breakfast		Water oz/ml
	Lunch	🏃	Exercise
	Dinner	🌙	Sleep h m
	Snacks	🧘	Stress Relief

Other

Sunday

Date   /   /

🍴		🗑	
	Breakfast		Water oz/ml
	Lunch	🏃	Exercise
	Dinner	🌙	Sleep h m
	Snacks	🧘	Stress Relief

Other

How am I feeling physically and mentally?

_____

_____

_____

_____

_____

_____

Challenges?

_____

_____

_____

_____

_____

_____

Achievements?

_____

_____

_____

_____

_____

_____

WEEK OF :   /   /   —   /   /

GOALS :
_____
_____
_____

Monday   Date   /   /

🍴	Breakfast		🗑 Water		oz/ml
	Lunch		🏃 Exercise		
	Dinner		🌙 Sleep	h	m
	Snacks		🧘 Stress Relief		

Other _____

Tuesday   Date   /   /

🍴	Breakfast		🗑 Water		oz/ml
	Lunch		🏃 Exercise		
	Dinner		🌙 Sleep	h	m
	Snacks		🧘 Stress Relief		

Other _____

Wednesday

Date / /

🍴	
Breakfast	🗑 Water ___ oz/ml
Lunch	🏃 Exercise
Dinner	🌙 Sleep ___ h ___ m
Snacks	🧘 Stress Relief

Other _____

Thursday

Date / /

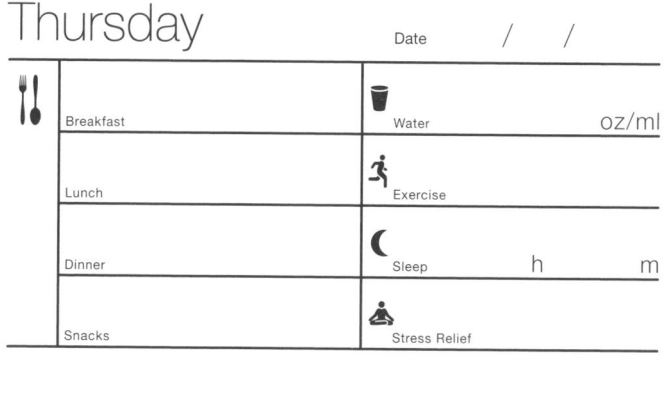

🍴	
Breakfast	🗑 Water ___ oz/ml
Lunch	🏃 Exercise
Dinner	🌙 Sleep ___ h ___ m
Snacks	🧘 Stress Relief

Other _____

Friday

Date / /

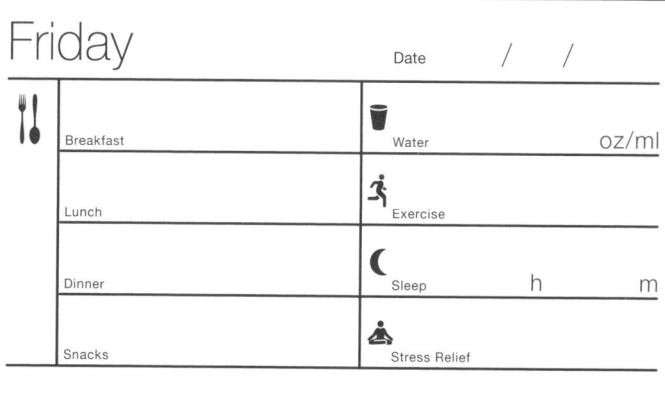

🍴	
Breakfast	🗑 Water ___ oz/ml
Lunch	🏃 Exercise
Dinner	🌙 Sleep ___ h ___ m
Snacks	🧘 Stress Relief

Other _____

Saturday

Date   /   /

Breakfast	Water oz/ml
Lunch	Exercise
Dinner	Sleep h m
Snacks	Stress Relief

Other _____

Sunday

Date   /   /

Breakfast	Water oz/ml
Lunch	Exercise
Dinner	Sleep h m
Snacks	Stress Relief

Other _____

How am I feeling physically and mentally?

Challenges?

Achievements?

WEEK OF :   /   /   —   /   /

GOALS :
_____
_____
_____

Monday   Date   /   /

🍴	Breakfast	🗑 Water	oz/ml
	Lunch	🏃 Exercise	
	Dinner	🌙 Sleep	h m
	Snacks	🧘 Stress Relief	

Other _____

Tuesday   Date   /   /

🍴	Breakfast	🗑 Water	oz/ml
	Lunch	🏃 Exercise	
	Dinner	🌙 Sleep	h m
	Snacks	🧘 Stress Relief	

Other _____

Wednesday

Date   /   /

🍴		
	Breakfast	🥤 Water oz/ml
	Lunch	🏃 Exercise
	Dinner	🌙 Sleep h m
	Snacks	🧘 Stress Relief

Other

Thursday

Date   /   /

🍴		
	Breakfast	🥤 Water oz/ml
	Lunch	🏃 Exercise
	Dinner	🌙 Sleep h m
	Snacks	🧘 Stress Relief

Other

Friday

Date   /   /

🍴		
	Breakfast	🥤 Water oz/ml
	Lunch	🏃 Exercise
	Dinner	🌙 Sleep h m
	Snacks	🧘 Stress Relief

Other

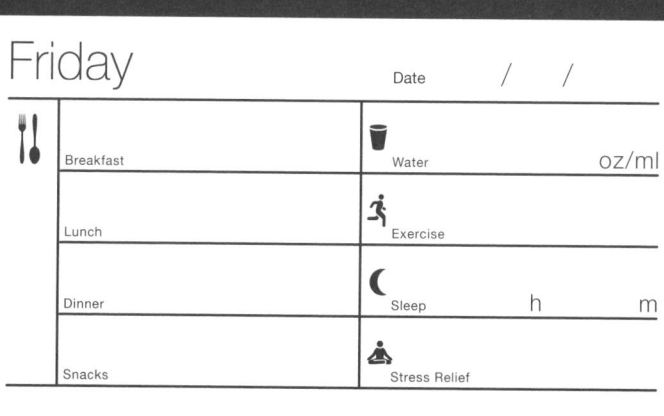

Saturday

Date   /   /

🍴 Breakfast		🗑 Water	oz/ml
Lunch		🏃 Exercise	
Dinner		🌙 Sleep	h m
Snacks		🧘 Stress Relief	

Other

Sunday

Date   /   /

🍴 Breakfast		🗑 Water	oz/ml
Lunch		🏃 Exercise	
Dinner		🌙 Sleep	h m
Snacks		🧘 Stress Relief	

Other

How am I feeling physically and mentally?

Challenges?

Achievements?

WEEK OF :   /   /   —   /   /

GOALS :
_____
_____
_____

Monday   Date   /   /

🍴	Breakfast	🥤	Water	oz/ml
	Lunch	🏃	Exercise	
	Dinner	🌙	Sleep	h m
	Snacks	🧘	Stress Relief	

Other _____

Tuesday   Date   /   /

🍴	Breakfast	🥤	Water	oz/ml
	Lunch	🏃	Exercise	
	Dinner	🌙	Sleep	h m
	Snacks	🧘	Stress Relief	

Other _____

Wednesday

Date   /   /

🍴			
	Breakfast	🗑 Water	oz/ml
	Lunch	🏃 Exercise	
	Dinner	🌙 Sleep	h m
	Snacks	🧘 Stress Relief	

Other _____

Thursday

Date   /   /

🍴			
	Breakfast	🗑 Water	oz/ml
	Lunch	🏃 Exercise	
	Dinner	🌙 Sleep	h m
	Snacks	🧘 Stress Relief	

Other _____

Friday

Date   /   /

🍴			
	Breakfast	🗑 Water	oz/ml
	Lunch	🏃 Exercise	
	Dinner	🌙 Sleep	h m
	Snacks	🧘 Stress Relief	

Other _____

Saturday

Date   /   /

Breakfast	Water	oz/ml
Lunch	Exercise	
Dinner	Sleep	h m
Snacks	Stress Relief	

Other

Sunday

Date   /   /

Breakfast	Water	oz/ml
Lunch	Exercise	
Dinner	Sleep	h m
Snacks	Stress Relief	

Other

How am I feeling physically and mentally?

Challenges?

Achievements?

WEEK OF :   /   /   —   /   /

GOALS :
_____
_____
_____

Monday   Date   /   /

Breakfast	Water	oz/ml
Lunch	Exercise	
Dinner	Sleep	h m
Snacks	Stress Relief	

Other _____

Tuesday   Date   /   /

Breakfast	Water	oz/ml
Lunch	Exercise	
Dinner	Sleep	h m
Snacks	Stress Relief	

Other _____

Wednesday

Date   /   /

🍴			
Breakfast		🗑 Water	oz/ml
Lunch		🏃 Exercise	
Dinner		🌙 Sleep	h m
Snacks		🧘 Stress Relief	

Other _____

Thursday

Date   /   /

🍴			
Breakfast		🗑 Water	oz/ml
Lunch		🏃 Exercise	
Dinner		🌙 Sleep	h m
Snacks		🧘 Stress Relief	

Other _____

Friday

Date   /   /

🍴			
Breakfast		🗑 Water	oz/ml
Lunch		🏃 Exercise	
Dinner		🌙 Sleep	h m
Snacks		🧘 Stress Relief	

Other _____

Saturday

Date   /   /

🍴			
	Breakfast	Water	oz/ml
	Lunch	Exercise	
	Dinner	Sleep h m	
	Snacks	Stress Relief	

Other

Sunday

Date   /   /

🍴			
	Breakfast	Water	oz/ml
	Lunch	Exercise	
	Dinner	Sleep h m	
	Snacks	Stress Relief	

Other

How am I feeling physically and mentally?

_____

_____

_____

_____

_____

_____

Challenges?

_____

_____

_____

_____

_____

_____

Achievements?

_____

_____

_____

_____

_____

_____

WEEK OF : / / — / /

GOALS :
_____
_____
_____

Monday

Date / /

Breakfast		Water	oz/ml
Lunch		Exercise	
Dinner		Sleep	h m
Snacks		Stress Relief	

Other _____

Tuesday

Date / /

Breakfast		Water	oz/ml
Lunch		Exercise	
Dinner		Sleep	h m
Snacks		Stress Relief	

Other _____

Wednesday

Date   /   /

🍴			
	Breakfast	🥛 Water	oz/ml
	Lunch	🏃 Exercise	
	Dinner	🌙 Sleep h m	
	Snacks	🧘 Stress Relief	

Other

Thursday

Date   /   /

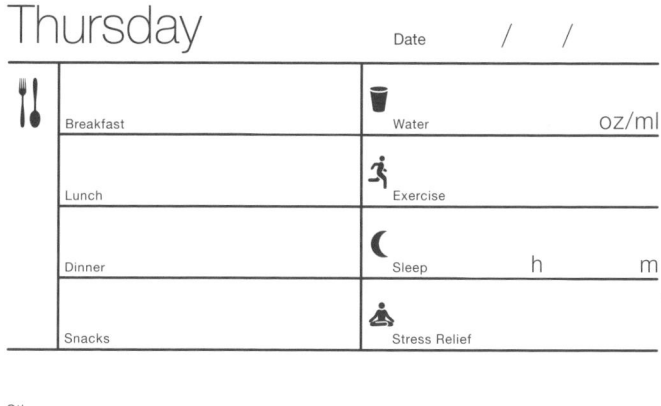

🍴			
	Breakfast	🥛 Water	oz/ml
	Lunch	🏃 Exercise	
	Dinner	🌙 Sleep h m	
	Snacks	🧘 Stress Relief	

Other

Friday

Date   /   /

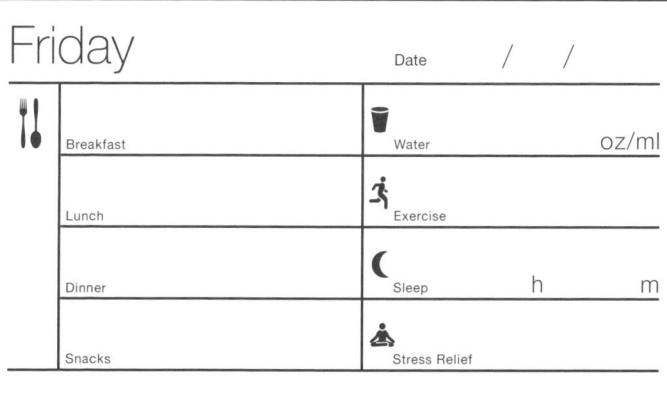

🍴			
	Breakfast	🥛 Water	oz/ml
	Lunch	🏃 Exercise	
	Dinner	🌙 Sleep h m	
	Snacks	🧘 Stress Relief	

Other

Saturday

Date   /   /

Breakfast	Water oz/ml
Lunch	Exercise
Dinner	Sleep h m
Snacks	Stress Relief

Other

Sunday

Date   /   /

Breakfast	Water oz/ml
Lunch	Exercise
Dinner	Sleep h m
Snacks	Stress Relief

Other

How am I feeling physically and mentally?

_____

_____

_____

_____

_____

_____

Challenges?

_____

_____

_____

_____

_____

_____

Achievements?

_____

_____

_____

_____

_____

_____

WEEK OF :   /   /   —   /   /

GOALS :

_____

_____

_____

Monday

Date   /   /

🍴	Breakfast		🥤 Water	oz/ml
	Lunch		🏃 Exercise	
	Dinner		🌙 Sleep	h m
	Snacks		🧘 Stress Relief	

Other _____

Tuesday

Date   /   /

🍴	Breakfast		🥤 Water	oz/ml
	Lunch		🏃 Exercise	
	Dinner		🌙 Sleep	h m
	Snacks		🧘 Stress Relief	

Other _____

Wednesday

Date ___ / ___ / ___

🍴	Breakfast	🗑 Water	oz/ml
	Lunch	🏃 Exercise	
	Dinner	🌙 Sleep	___ h ___ m
	Snacks	🧘 Stress Relief	

Other _____

Thursday

Date ___ / ___ / ___

🍴	Breakfast	🗑 Water	oz/ml
	Lunch	🏃 Exercise	
	Dinner	🌙 Sleep	___ h ___ m
	Snacks	🧘 Stress Relief	

Other _____

Friday

Date ___ / ___ / ___

🍴	Breakfast	🗑 Water	oz/ml
	Lunch	🏃 Exercise	
	Dinner	🌙 Sleep	___ h ___ m
	Snacks	🧘 Stress Relief	

Other _____

Saturday

Date   /   /

Breakfast	Water oz/ml
Lunch	Exercise
Dinner	Sleep h m
Snacks	Stress Relief

Other

Sunday

Date   /   /

Breakfast	Water oz/ml
Lunch	Exercise
Dinner	Sleep h m
Snacks	Stress Relief

Other

How am I feeling physically and mentally?

Challenges?

Achievements?

WEEK OF :   /   /   —   /   /

GOALS :
_____
_____
_____

Monday
Date   /   /

🍴
Breakfast	🗑 Water	oz/ml
Lunch	🏃 Exercise	
Dinner	🌙 Sleep	h m
Snacks	🧘 Stress Relief	

Other _____

Tuesday
Date   /   /

🍴
Breakfast	🗑 Water	oz/ml
Lunch	🏃 Exercise	
Dinner	🌙 Sleep	h m
Snacks	🧘 Stress Relief	

Other _____

Wednesday

Date   /   /

Breakfast	Water oz/ml
Lunch	Exercise
Dinner	Sleep h m
Snacks	Stress Relief

Other

Thursday

Date   /   /

Breakfast	Water oz/ml
Lunch	Exercise
Dinner	Sleep h m
Snacks	Stress Relief

Other

Friday

Date   /   /

Breakfast	Water oz/ml
Lunch	Exercise
Dinner	Sleep h m
Snacks	Stress Relief

Other

Saturday

Date   /   /

Breakfast	Water	oz/ml
Lunch	Exercise	
Dinner	Sleep	h m
Snacks	Stress Relief	

Other

Sunday

Date   /   /

Breakfast	Water	oz/ml
Lunch	Exercise	
Dinner	Sleep	h m
Snacks	Stress Relief	

Other

How am I feeling physically and mentally?

Challenges?

Achievements?

WEEK OF :   /   /   —   /   /

GOALS :
_____
_____
_____

Monday

Date   /   /

Breakfast		Water		oz/ml
Lunch		Exercise		
Dinner		Sleep	h	m
Snacks		Stress Relief		

Other

Tuesday

Date   /   /

Breakfast		Water		oz/ml
Lunch		Exercise		
Dinner		Sleep	h	m
Snacks		Stress Relief		

Other

Wednesday

Date   /   /

!			Water	oz/ml
	Breakfast			
	Lunch		Exercise	
	Dinner		Sleep	h m
	Snacks		Stress Relief	

Other _____

Thursday

Date   /   /

!			Water	oz/ml
	Breakfast			
	Lunch		Exercise	
	Dinner		Sleep	h m
	Snacks		Stress Relief	

Other _____

Friday

Date   /   /

!			Water	oz/ml
	Breakfast			
	Lunch		Exercise	
	Dinner		Sleep	h m
	Snacks		Stress Relief	

Other _____

Saturday

Date   /   /

Breakfast	Water oz/ml
Lunch	Exercise
Dinner	Sleep h m
Snacks	Stress Relief

Other

Sunday

Date   /   /

Breakfast	Water oz/ml
Lunch	Exercise
Dinner	Sleep h m
Snacks	Stress Relief

Other

How am I feeling physically and mentally?

_____
_____
_____
_____
_____
_____

Challenges?

_____
_____
_____
_____
_____
_____

Achievements?

_____
_____
_____
_____
_____
_____

WEEK OF :   /   /   —   /   /

GOALS :
_____
_____
_____

Monday   Date   /   /

🍴 | Breakfast | 🗑 Water | oz/ml
| Lunch | 🏃 Exercise |
| Dinner | 🌙 Sleep | h | m
| Snacks | 🧘 Stress Relief |

Other _____

Tuesday   Date   /   /

🍴 | Breakfast | 🗑 Water | oz/ml
| Lunch | 🏃 Exercise |
| Dinner | 🌙 Sleep | h | m
| Snacks | 🧘 Stress Relief |

Other _____

Wednesday

Date ___ / ___ / ___

🍴	Breakfast		🗑 Water	oz/ml
	Lunch		🏃 Exercise	
	Dinner		🌙 Sleep	h m
	Snacks		🧘 Stress Relief	

Other _____

Thursday

Date ___ / ___ / ___

🍴	Breakfast		🗑 Water	oz/ml
	Lunch		🏃 Exercise	
	Dinner		🌙 Sleep	h m
	Snacks		🧘 Stress Relief	

Other _____

Friday

Date ___ / ___ / ___

🍴	Breakfast		🗑 Water	oz/ml
	Lunch		🏃 Exercise	
	Dinner		🌙 Sleep	h m
	Snacks		🧘 Stress Relief	

Other _____

Saturday

Date   /   /

Breakfast		Water	oz/ml
Lunch		Exercise	
Dinner		Sleep	h m
Snacks		Stress Relief	

Other

Sunday

Date   /   /

Breakfast		Water	oz/ml
Lunch		Exercise	
Dinner		Sleep	h m
Snacks		Stress Relief	

Other

How am I feeling physically and mentally?

_____

_____

_____

_____

_____

_____

Challenges?

_____

_____

_____

_____

_____

_____

Achievements?

_____

_____

_____

_____

_____

_____

WEEK OF :   /   /   —   /   /

GOALS :

_____

_____

_____

Monday

Date   /   /

Breakfast	Water	oz/ml
Lunch	Exercise	
Dinner	Sleep	h m
Snacks	Stress Relief	

Other _____

Tuesday

Date   /   /

Breakfast	Water	oz/ml
Lunch	Exercise	
Dinner	Sleep	h m
Snacks	Stress Relief	

Other _____

Wednesday

Date   /   /

Breakfast		Water	oz/ml
Lunch		Exercise	
Dinner		Sleep	h m
Snacks		Stress Relief	

Other _____

Thursday

Date   /   /

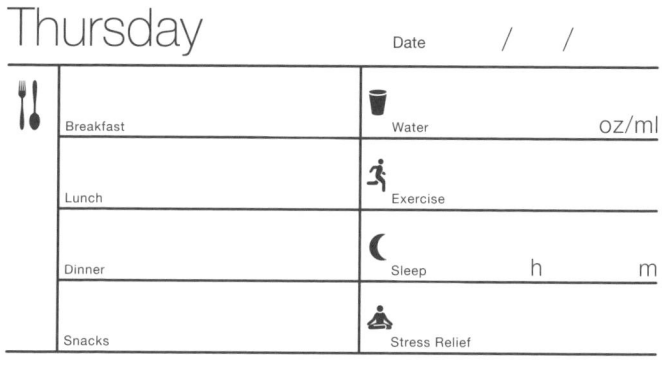

Breakfast		Water	oz/ml
Lunch		Exercise	
Dinner		Sleep	h m
Snacks		Stress Relief	

Other _____

Friday

Date   /   /

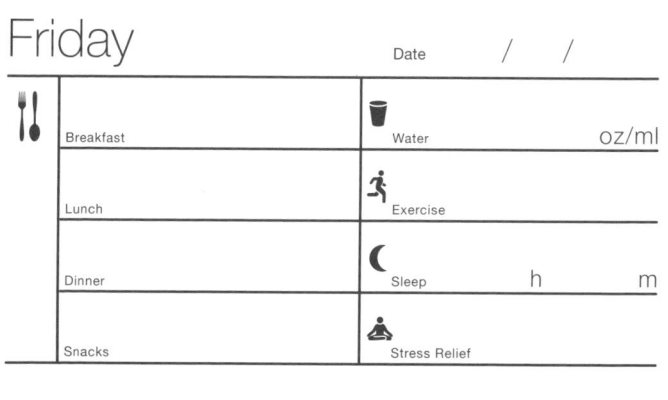

Breakfast		Water	oz/ml
Lunch		Exercise	
Dinner		Sleep	h m
Snacks		Stress Relief	

Other _____

Saturday

Date   /   /

Breakfast	Water oz/ml
Lunch	Exercise
Dinner	Sleep h m
Snacks	Stress Relief

Other

Sunday

Date   /   /

Breakfast	Water oz/ml
Lunch	Exercise
Dinner	Sleep h m
Snacks	Stress Relief

Other

How am I feeling physically and mentally?

_____

_____

_____

_____

_____

_____

Challenges?

_____

_____

_____

_____

_____

_____

Achievements?

_____

_____

_____

_____

_____

_____

WEEK OF :   /   /   —   /   /

GOALS :
_____
_____
_____

Monday   Date   /   /

🍴			
	Breakfast	🗑 Water	oz/ml
	Lunch	🏃 Exercise	
	Dinner	🌙 Sleep	h m
	Snacks	🧘 Stress Relief	

Other _____

Tuesday   Date   /   /

🍴			
	Breakfast	🗑 Water	oz/ml
	Lunch	🏃 Exercise	
	Dinner	🌙 Sleep	h m
	Snacks	🧘 Stress Relief	

Other _____

Wednesday

Date   /   /

🍴			
	Breakfast	🗑 Water	oz/ml
	Lunch	🏃 Exercise	
	Dinner	🌙 Sleep	h m
	Snacks	🧘 Stress Relief	

Other

Thursday

Date   /   /

🍴			
	Breakfast	🗑 Water	oz/ml
	Lunch	🏃 Exercise	
	Dinner	🌙 Sleep	h m
	Snacks	🧘 Stress Relief	

Other

Friday

Date   /   /

🍴			
	Breakfast	🗑 Water	oz/ml
	Lunch	🏃 Exercise	
	Dinner	🌙 Sleep	h m
	Snacks	🧘 Stress Relief	

Other

Saturday

Date   /   /

Breakfast	Water	oz/ml
Lunch	Exercise	
Dinner	Sleep h m	
Snacks	Stress Relief	

Other

Sunday

Date   /   /

Breakfast	Water	oz/ml
Lunch	Exercise	
Dinner	Sleep h m	
Snacks	Stress Relief	

Other

How am I feeling physically and mentally?

Challenges?

Achievements?

WEEK OF :   /   /   —   /   /

GOALS :
_____
_____
_____

Monday

Date   /   /

🍴				
	Breakfast	🥤 Water		oz/ml
	Lunch	🏃 Exercise		
	Dinner	🌙 Sleep	h	m
	Snacks	🧘 Stress Relief		

Other _____

Tuesday

Date   /   /

🍴				
	Breakfast	🥤 Water		oz/ml
	Lunch	🏃 Exercise		
	Dinner	🌙 Sleep	h	m
	Snacks	🧘 Stress Relief		

Other _____

Wednesday

Date ___ / ___ / ___

🍴		
	Breakfast	🗑 Water _____ oz/ml
	Lunch	🏃 Exercise
	Dinner	🌙 Sleep ___ h ___ m
	Snacks	🧘 Stress Relief

Other _____

Thursday

Date ___ / ___ / ___

🍴		
	Breakfast	🗑 Water _____ oz/ml
	Lunch	🏃 Exercise
	Dinner	🌙 Sleep ___ h ___ m
	Snacks	🧘 Stress Relief

Other _____

Friday

Date ___ / ___ / ___

🍴		
	Breakfast	🗑 Water _____ oz/ml
	Lunch	🏃 Exercise
	Dinner	🌙 Sleep ___ h ___ m
	Snacks	🧘 Stress Relief

Other _____

Saturday

Date   /   /

🍴	Breakfast	🗑 Water		oz/ml
	Lunch	🏃 Exercise		
	Dinner	🌙 Sleep	h	m
	Snacks	🧘 Stress Relief		

Other

Sunday

Date   /   /

🍴	Breakfast	🗑 Water		oz/ml
	Lunch	🏃 Exercise		
	Dinner	🌙 Sleep	h	m
	Snacks	🧘 Stress Relief		

Other

How am I feeling physically and mentally?

_____

_____

_____

_____

_____

_____

Challenges?

_____

_____

_____

_____

_____

Achievements?

_____

_____

_____

_____

_____

_____

Notes

Notes

Notes